BIOCHEMIC TISSUE SALTS

A natural way to prevent and cure illness

BIOCHEMIC TISSUE SALTS

A natural way to prevent and cure illness

Andrew Stanway MB, MRCP

THORSONS PUBLISHING GROUP
Wellingborough, Northamptonshire
—————— · ——————
Rochester, Vermont

First published by Van Dyke Books Ltd. 1982
This edition published 1987

© Andrew Stanway 1982

British Library Cataloguing in Publication Data

Stanway, Andrew
Biochemic tissue salts: a natural way to
prevent and cure illness.
1. Medicine, Biochemic   2. Salts
I. Title
615.8'54   RZ412

ISBN 0-7225-1156-6

Printed and bound in Great Britain

1 3 5 7 9 10 8 6 4 2

CONTENTS

PART THREE: SELECTING A REMEDY

Acknowledgments

I should like to thank the following, without whose help the book would not have been possible:

Dr P. Gilbert; New Era Laboratories; and Dr M. Sian of Charing Cross Hospital, London.

Note to reader

Before following the self-help advice given in this book, readers are urged to give careful consideration to the nature of their particular health problem and to consult a competent physician if in any doubt. This book should not be regarded as a substitute for professional medical treatment and, whilst every care is taken to ensure the accuracy of the content, the author and the publishers cannot accept legal responsibility for any problem arising out of the experimentation with the methods described.

About the author

Dr Andrew Stanway MB, MRCP qualified in medicine in 1968 and practised on the Medical Professorial Unit at King's College Hospital, London. After 3 years of medical practice (during which time he became a Member of the Royal College of Physicians) he went full-time into medical writing and film making. He has spent the last 20 years writing about medicine for the public and promoting health education.

He lives in Surrey with his wife and three children.

PART ONE

INTRODUCTION

INTRODUCTION

We are living in exciting times—people are becoming more health conscious and at the same time more aware that they can influence their own health both by preventing illness and by treating simple things themselves. Along with this trend is the realization that perhaps there are answers to health care other than those provided by the conventional medical establishment. Alternative or complementary medical therapies are used more than ever and books abound on the subject. People in general are waking up to the fact that western technological medicine cannot hope to answer all their health needs.

Only a couple of centuries ago medicine was a blend of art, science, myth, magic and superstition. Today it is overwhelmingly a scientific extension of western 20th century technology. The other facets have been ignored, overruled or so debased as to render them useless. This is a shame because man is so obviously not a mere collection of parts and to treat him as such is to reduce him to a kind of machine. Reductionist theories of medicine are at last becoming less popular, at least with some of the public, who simply don't believe that a deep understanding of the intimate workings of the cell and its constituents is either necessary or desirable in treating the vast majority of common ailments.

People have always wanted alternative forms of medical therapy to those which are readily available but today in the West the need is apparently greater than ever. This has probably come about for five main reasons: people see orthodox therapies failing in certain conditions (especially chronic ones) and find this hard to accept; many are afraid of western medical treatment with its operations and drug side-effects; some people have religious or philosophical arguments against certain western practices; there is a growing minority of people of all ages who feel it is time to protest about what *is* available; and lastly there always has been, and hopefully always will be, a proportion of the population who simply wants to be different and to experiment and this extends to the kind of medical care they demand. But whatever the reason for choosing alternative or unorthodox therapies, the starting point is the same—an ill person.

Self-medication, a popular answer for common ailments

Many people do nothing at all for minor aches, pains and everyday ailments, yet they improve. This is a fact to bear in mind from the start; there are large numbers of complaints that get better by themselves whatever action the sufferer takes. There is a step between doing nothing at all and seeking outside help and that is to try to cure oneself. Millions of people the world over do this every day: traditional cures for colds and 'flu abound and each nation and even regions within nations develop their own remedies for common ailments. 'Self-medication' is encouraged by pharmaceutical and other companies and all over the world there are patent medicines available which promise great things in return for a small outlay.

When a person seeks medical help he is usually suffering from one of four groups of conditions. The condition may be self-limiting as I've already mentioned; it may be chronic, with an uneven succession of partial recoveries and relapses; it may be of psychological or environmental origin (caused by difficulties within the family and in interpersonal relationships, work trouble, poor housing, money problems, and so on); or it might actually be an acute medical condition.

All of these people are *ill* and will undoubtedly benefit from some sort of treatment. Those with a self-limiting illness will get better anyway: the chronically ill can be offered symptomatic relief but know that their condition fluctuates and that their improvement might not have been brought about by the treatment; the psychologically-based group needs understanding and help (much of which need not necessarily, or even ideally, come from a doctor); and the last group will really need modern western medicine.

The trouble is that most people imagine that doctors spend their time seeing and curing this last group. In reality this group makes up less than 20 per cent of those going to general practitioners. The other 80 per cent fall into the other three groups and simply don't *need* western medicine *per se*. Many of them would fare just as well if they didn't live in the sophisticated western world.

Unfortunately, a person who is 'ill' and chooses to go to his doctor has only one of two therapeutic choices open to him. Either he can take the medication his doctor offers or he can do nothing. With the loss of the tonics and other harmless medications so popular with the older generation of general practitioners, today's practitioner has little to offer that isn't a powerful pharmaceutical agent with actual (or potential) side-effects. In practice this means that substantial proportions of all the medicines prescribed and dispensed at enormous cost to the nation never get swallowed, often because the patient is unhappy about side-effects he has heard about, can't tolerate those that do occur, or is worried about other side-effects he (and the medical profession) don't yet know about. Many an 'old-fashioned' family doctor had his own special brand of tablets—often effective, always harmless, made up by himself in the practice—which, when given with kind and loving care, had the effects he and his patient desired. Alas, there are few, if any, such products available today, much to the chagrin of many doctors old and young.

The power of the placebo

Because the medical profession is not supplying the public with what they want in this area, others have stepped into the gap. Increasing numbers of people appreciate the value of health food shops which are opening in large numbers each year. Here they find 'health' products which are safe, often with a very long history and based on natural remedies. They take these instead of the tonics doctors used to prescribe but there is little doubt that many such products also have therapeutic effects as well as a potent placebo ('dummy') effect.

This all fits in well with the current trend for 'naturalness' in the western world. Manufacturers of everything from bath cleaners to pharmaceutical products are cashing in on the 'back to nature' trend in society. The growth of interest in health foods and other do-it-yourself health products is simply a part of this movement. It would be foolish to write off the health movement as a cranky, middle class fad because there is every sign that it is here to stay, involves all classes and types of people, makes sense in most cases and is being increasingly validated by orthodox scientific medicine.

The reason this has come about is that the new breed of 'scientific' doctor believes that he should use only medications which have been proven to have pharmaceutical effects and have been shown to be tolerably safe. This unfortunately ignores the fact that placebo tables have a measurable effect in between 30 and 50 per cent of those taking them for very real symptoms. Even some so-called 'real' pharmaceutical preparations are effective in only a small proportion of people and some preparations have adverse effects on a significant proportion, so reducing the numbers that can take them at all.

All of this, it seems to many, leaves the way wide open for a safe, easy-to-use system of medication that can often do good and does so at a very low cost. Biochemic Tissue Salts are such remedies and deserve far greater recognition than they have so far received.

PART TWO

BIOCHEMICS

WHAT IS BIOCHEMICS?

The word 'biochemics' is derived from the Greek word for 'life' (*bios*) and 'chemistry' and is a branch of medicine which concerns itself with chemical changes that take place in living organisms. Biochemistry is the modern study of such functions but *biochemics* is a more restricted study of certain specific chemicals in the body. Biochemistry is a whole scientific discipline but biochemics is a specific system of medicine devised by one man, Dr W. H. Schuessler, just over a century ago—long before modern biochemistry as we know it got off the ground.

Of all the systems of medical thought and treatment over the centuries, few can compete with biochemics for simplicity. By today's standards it seems almost too simple and there are those who would like to see it enlarged in its compass and complexity to take into account new physiological and biochemical knowledge about the body and its constituents including the salts and trace elements. Having said this though, there is no reason to write it off *because* it is so simple.

It had long been held that inorganic salts normally present in the human body were vital to its healthy functioning but it wasn't until 1832 in Stapt's *Archiv* that the following was written: 'All the essential component parts of the human body are great remedies . . . All the constituents of the human body act in such organs principally when they have a function.' Rudolph Virchow, the father of pathology, discovered that the body was composed of millions of tiny cells, each one composed of organic (living) and inorganic (non-living) substances which work in perfect balance and with this new knowledge biochemics began to make sense to the new breed of scientist.

In 1873 though, when a German doctor of medicine from Oldenburg—William H. Schuessler—began to publish a series of papers on the subject, body tissue salts began to be taken seriously both in nature and as therapeutic agents.

Over the years Schuessler proved, to his satisfaction, that certain mineral (or as he called them 'tissue') salts were vitally important to the healthy functioning of the human body. He reasoned (sensibly for that time) that the vast majority of the inorganic salts of the body were in the bones. What he couldn't measure, although he knew they were important, were the concentrations of inorganic salts in the body's other structures and fluids. In spite of this very real handicap he was able to decide upon the 12 tissue salts that were, in his opinion, vital to cell function.

WHAT ARE THE TISSUE SALTS?

The twelve Schuessler tissue salts are:
1. Calcium Fluoride (*Calc. Fluor.*)
2. Calcium Phosphate (*Calc. Phos.*)
3. Calcium Sulphate (*Calc. Sulph.*)
4. Iron Phosphate (*Ferr. Phos.*)
5. Potassium Chloride (*Kali. Mur.*)
6. Potassium Phosphate (*Kali. Phos.*)
7. Potassium Sulphate (*Kali. Sulph.*)
8. Magnesium Phosphate (*Mag. Phos.*)
9. Sodium Chloride (*Nat. Mur.*)
10. Sodium Phosphate (*Nat. Phos.*)
11. Sodium Sulphate (*Nat. Sulph.*)
12. Silicon Dioxide (*Silica*)

The names in brackets are the shortened Latin equivalent names. Those who use the tissue salts point out that it is really incorrect to use the English names because, for example, sodium chloride (table salt) is simply crystalline salt whereas *Nat. Mur.* is the homoeopathically prepared, biochemically active equivalent. In other words common table salt, specially prepared in a homoeopathic way, becomes *Nat. Mur.* and takes on properties which are over and above those of common salt. This is in essence the principle of biochemic tissue salts and their use in everyday therapy.

Today some practitioners and very large numbers of the public use combinations of the salts as medical remedies because, they argue, Schuessler himself suggested that combinations be used together in certain situations. The major producer in the UK (New Era Laboratories) has produced a whole series of combinations which, they claim, have greater biological activity and are easier to take than the same salts used individually in certain conditions.

These combination therapies are named alphabetically as Combinations A–S and have different therapeutic uses. They contain the following tissue salts combined in a single tablet:

Combination	Tissue salts contained
A	Ferr. Phos., Kali. Phos., Mag. Phos.
B	Calc. Phos., Kali. Phos., Ferr. Phos.
C	Mag. Phos., Nat. Phos., Nat. Sulph., Silica
D	Kali. Mur., Kali Sulph., Calc. Sulph., Silica
E	Calc. Phos., Mag. Phos., Nat. Phos., Nat. Sulph.
F	Kali. Phos., Mag. Phos., Nat. Mur., Silica
G	Calc. Fluor., Calc. Phos., Kali. Phos., Nat. Mur.
H	Mag. Phos., Nat. Mur., Silica
I	Ferr. Phos., Kali. Sulph. Mag. Phos.
J	Ferr. Phos., Kali. Sulph., Nat. Mur.
K	Kali. Sulph., Nat. Mur., Silica
L	Calc. Fluor., Ferr. Phos., Nat. Mur.
M	Calc. Phos., Kali. Mur., Nat. Phos., Nat. Sulph.
N	Calc. Phos., Kali. Mur., Kali. Phos., Mag. Phos.
P	Calc. Fluor., Calc. Phos., Kali. Phos., Mag. Phos.
Q	Ferr. Phos., Kali. Mur., Kali. Sulph., Nat. Mur.
R	Calc. Fluor., Calc. Phos., Ferr. Phos., Mag. Phos., Silica.
S	Kali. Mur., Nat. Phos., Nat. Sulph.

These combinations and their uses are described in more detail on page 32.

Schuessler studied and defined the function of each of the 12 basic tissue salts and detailed very carefully the disorders he thought would arise if any was deficient or present in reduced concentrations in the body. In doing this he built up his five principles of biochemics which today's practitioners still use as a guide.

1. Disease does not occur if cell metabolism is normal.

2. Cell metabolism is in turn normal if cell nutrition is adequate.

3. Nutritional substances are either of an organic or inorganic nature as far as the body is concerned.

4. The ability of the body cells to assimilate and to excrete and further to utilize nutritional material is impaired if there is a deficiency in the inorganic material (tissue salt) constituent of tissues.

5. Adequate cell nutrition may be restored and cellular metabolism normalized by supplying the required tissue salts to the organism in a finely divided assimilable form.

Strange though it may seem, this rather ordinary (by today's standards) assertion that inorganic salts were valuable to the body in specific ways caught on in a big way. Schuessler's original work was the subject of 56 editions over the years and was being revised and improved upon right up to his death in 1898.

THE SPREAD OF BIOCHEMICS

All Schuessler's original work was, of course, in German but it was translated into English by H. C. G. Luyties, of St Louis, Missouri, who visited Dr Schuessler in Germany on many occasions. Various other English language translations of Schuessler's works appeared on both sides of the Atlantic and today there are many for the interested reader to choose from.

Biochemic tissue salts were used by many doctors early this century in the UK. One of the main pioneers was Dr Henry Gilbert, founder of the British Biochemic Association in 1911. His son, Dr Peter Gilbert, is still practising biochemics in London today. Gilbert senior was a close colleague of Dr Hensel, a disciple of Schuessler and with such an auspicious pedigree Gilbert started the School of Biochemics in London. He ran this as a way of training doctors in the Schuessler method and was later joined by his son Peter who taught and practised at the school for many years. With the death of Gilbert senior in 1962 and ever-escalating costs the school had to close. At its height, around the First World War, there were more than 50 doctors practising biochemic therapy in the UK but today Dr Peter Gilbert is probably the only remaining full-time practitioner in the country and he has greatly extended and modified Schuessler's original work. Even his father had extended the number of remedies from 12 to about 70 and Peter Gilbert uses many more. The number of possible combinations is enormous. This contrasts with Schuessler's own desire that the therapy be kept as simple as possible—a considerably easier and more achievable task in the chemically straightforward days of over 100 years ago. It is said that Schuessler even wanted to *reduce* the number of tissue salts from 12 to make therapy simpler still. This never caught on in practice and with the growth of knowledge about biochemistry it is unlikely that the system will ever be simplified.

THE RELATIONSHIP BETWEEN BIOCHEMICS AND HOMOEOPATHY

Biochemics is really a branch of homoeopathy only in the sense that the tissue salts are produced in the same way as are homoeopathic remedies. Most of the 12 Schuessler tissue salts were included in the list of standard homoeopathic remedies many years before Schuessler himself expounded his biochemic therapy and many of today's homoeopaths use them in their day-to-day work.

Undoubtedly Schuessler was influenced by Hahnemann, the father of homoeopathy, and should perhaps best be seen as a key figure in the historical development of homoeopathic medicine. Others were Hahnemann (who 'invented' homoeopathy) and Rudolph Steiner, the father of anthroposophical medicine. The big difference between most homoeopaths and those who use biochemic remedies is that homoeopaths use almost any active substance in minute concentrations, provided that it produces the same clinical signs and symptoms as the disease it is being used to treat. Biochemic therapists, however, use only those inorganic salts that occur naturally in the body: they use nothing else.

Having said this though, both branches of medicine have a lot in common. They rely on the patient's symptoms as their guide for remedy selection and use the remedies in minute doses. Dr Schuessler said in his book *An Abridged Therapy*, 'Whenever small doses are mentioned one usually at once thinks of Homoeopathy; my therapy, however, is not Homoeopathic, for it is not founded in the law of similarity, but on the physiologic-chemical process which takes place in the human organism. By my method of cure the disturbances occurring in the motion of the molecules of the inorganic substances in the human body are directly equalized by means of homogeneous substances, while Homoeopathy attains its curative ends in an indirect way by means of heterogeneous substances.

'Some have averred that these remedies, as Silica and Calcium Phosphate, etc. which had already been used by physicians before biochemistry was established, are on that account not biochemical remedies. It would be just as correct or rather incorrect to assert that all remedies used before Hahnemann belong exclusively to allopathy.

'But the truth of the matter is:

'The principle according to which a remedy is selected stamps its impress upon it. A remedy selected according to the principle of similars is a homoeopathic remedy, but a remedy which is homogeneous with the mineral substances of the organism, and the use of which is founded on physiological chemistry, is a biochemic remedy.'

Today, many homoeopaths, both lay and medically qualified, use the tissue salts, though to be fair there is considerable disagreement between homoeopaths and others about the best way to use them. This inter-professional disagreement does nothing to take away from the fact that the tissue salts produce provable results in thousands of satisfied patients.

HOW ARE THEY MADE?

Dr Schuessler made his remedies using the homoeopathic principle of trituration. In this, one part of the active salt is diluted with 9 parts of milk sugar (lactose) and ground gently. One part of this mixture is then taken and diluted with a further 9 parts of lactose and the process repeated until the salt has undergone 6 successive dilutions and grindings. At this stage the original salt is present in a concentration of 1 part per million of lactose but has, it is claimed, become 'potentised'. Although many potentisations (numbers of serial dilutions and grindings) can be used— and indeed were at the turn of the century—experience has found that 6 dilutions and grindings (6x) is the most effective therapeutically and safest for the public to use without professional guidance. It is possible to potentise Schuessler salts more but they can then be too powerful.

The final lactose and tissue salt mixture is gently 'moulded' into a very friable tablet that dissolves under the tongue in about 5 seconds, ensuring immediate absorption into the bloodstream. It is only because of the physical properties of lactose that this is possible.

The method that Schuessler used is still used today by the leading manufacturers of tissue salts but they have automated the process and use very large quantities of everything because they are producing millions of doses at a time.

At the laboratories of the UK's foremost producer of tissue salts, they faithfully adhere to the principles of the Schuessler method. Porcelain spheres roll for hours inside porcelain tubs of lactose and the active ingredients as the serial triturations are made. The production is carried out under the strictest levels of control as for pharmaceutical preparations: in fact the regulations of the Department of Health are strictly applied. Batches are tested by full-time biochemists and quality control is constantly monitored. Because the amount of active ingredients in each tablet is so tiny this calls for great care and skill.

From what has been said so far it can be seen that a tablet of a tissue salt is composed almost entirely of lactose. Because of this it is important to be sure that you are not intolerant of lactose before taking the tablets. You will probably already know if you are because you will have had unpleasant abdominal symptoms after drinking cows' milk in the past and will probably not now be drinking it at all anyway. This intolerance comes about as a result of an acquired deficiency of lactase, the vital intestinal enzyme needed to deal with lactose in the gut. People with lactose intolerance form the only proven group of people who cannot tolerate tissue salt therapy, though of course it is not the salts themselves that cause their problem.

WHAT DO THE TISSUE SALTS DO IN THE BODY?

Most books on biochemics have page after page of claimed activities for each salt with all kinds of pseudo-scientific jargon to back them up. There really is no excuse for this today when biochemistry is so sophisticated and the effects of the salts' constituents are to a great extent known and proved.

I shall now describe the action in the body of each part of the 12 tissue salts and in the next section we shall see how they might produce their activities at a level which is not explicable simply on 'chemical' grounds.

In general, the minerals in the body have five main known functions:

1. They are components of enzymes.
2. They are essential for nerve impulse transmission.
3. They carry oxygen.
4. They form the building blocks for bones and teeth.
5. They are components of hormones.

The minerals that are present in largest quantities in the body function mainly as components of bone or control the body's fluid balance by virtue of their concentration. The salts most involved in these activities are calcium, phosphorus, sodium chloride, potassium chloride and magnesium.

The inorganic substances to be found in the tissue salts (and their combinations) are:

Calcium	Potassium
Fluorine	Chloride
Phosphate	Magnesium
Sulphate	Silicon
Iron	Sodium

When Schuessler put forward his system of medicine and salt therapy these were the only chemical substances considered to be important. Today, however, with infinitely more sophisticated analytical methods, we know that there are whole hosts of other inorganic chemical substances that are essential for the normal functioning of the body. These substances, present only in tiny concentrations in the body, are known as trace elements, because only traces of them are necessary for life. Such traces simply couldn't have been detected by Schuessler's contemporaries but are no less important for all that.

First let's look at the major minerals.

1. Calcium and 2. Phosphorus

These two are considered together because they are so often found together in the body and often act together too. They are the most abundant minerals in the body and occur mainly in the skeleton. A 70kg (11 stone) man will have about 0.9-1.4kg (2-3 lb) of calcium and between 0.5 and 0.8kg (1.2 and 1.7 lb) of phosphorus in his body. Ninety per cent of the calcium is in the bones and teeth, but calcium and phosphorus aren't simply present in a static form in the bones and teeth: there is a considerable exchange every day between the skeleton and the fluids surrounding the body's cells. It has been calculated that 700mg of calcium enters and leaves the skeleton every day in an adult.

Bones act as reservoirs for calcium and phosphorus, where they are stored in crystalline forms. When the dietary intake of these minerals is inadequate to meet the body's requirements, the bones supply them so as to maintain a normal, physiological balance. Once these stores are used up, the body actually breaks down bone itself, so crucial are these substances to its functioning. A shortage of calcium and phosphorus can occur if too little is eaten in the diet but a deficiency can also occur even in the presence of an adequate dietary intake if there is a shortage of vitamin D—the vitamin essential for calcium metabolism.

As we have seen, the vast majority of calcium is tied up in bones and teeth but there is a small but vital amount in the blood and extra-cellular fluids. Though the quantity is small it is essential for life because it controls the excitability of nerves and muscles. A reduction of body calcium produces a condition known as tetany in which nerves controlling movement become ultra-sensitive to stimuli. The hands, face and feet are especially likely to be affected. The muscles lose tone and become flaccid and calcium is required to cure the condition.

Calcium is also essential in the process of blood clotting and for the normal function of heart muscles (and indeed all muscles); for the functioning of the 'cement substances' that hold body cells together; and for the functioning of various membranes in the body. It is also of proven value in such essential processes as lactation, nerve conduction and the release of hormones and it antagonizes the effects of magnesium in some enzymatic processes.

Calcium outside the bones and teeth is kept at a remarkably constant level. Over a period of 24 hours it fluctuates less than 3 per cent in the plasma—a state which is maintained by hormonal control.

Calcium may also help control cholesterol levels. One trial found that the mineral probably acts by inhibiting cholesterol absorption from the intestine.

Phosphorus, as well as playing a role in skeletal formation, structure and metabolism is also involved in many other vital metabolic processes. It is present as soluble phosphate in cells and fluids where it forms (with chloride) the main negatively charged group of ions (called anions), which neutralize the positively charged ions (cations) such as sodium, potassium, calcium and magnesium. Phosphorus is also present in proteins, fats and carbohydrates. It is essential for the conversion of glucose to glycogen and for the breakdown of glucose to produce energy in the cells. The B-complex vitamins can exert their beneficial effects only when combined with phosphorus.

It is difficult to be short of phosphorus unless you're taking a lot of non-absorbed antacids but you can easily consume too much phosphorus in the form of soft drinks and processed foods, many of which are high in phosphates.

3. Magnesium

This salt is closely related to calcium and phosphorus in its locations in the body and in its functions. Most is present in the bones which act as its reservoir. At a cellular level there is a considerable difference between magnesium, calcium and phosphate.

Calcium is present outside the cells whereas magnesium is mainly found inside. The gradient that this produces is partly responsible for the difference in the electrical potential that exists across cell membranes and which helps to transmit impulses to muscles. A magnesium deficiency in man produces excitability, tremors, convulsions and depression.

Doctors used to scoff at the thought of magnesium deficiencies but, with increased amounts of processed foods being consumed, it is quite possible that many people are actually short of magnesium, if only subclinically.

There is an interesting link between heart disease and magnesium. It has been found in several parts of the world that heart attacks are less common in hard water areas. There is some evidence that an increased magnesium intake protects heart muscle against this hazard.

The body tends to lose magnesium with gastro-intestinal and kidney diseases—prolonged diarrhoea is especially likely to deplete the body of this vital mineral. Very low levels occur in chronic alcoholics and it is certain that heavy drinkers need more of this mineral than normal people.

It has also been found that vitamin B_6 and magnesium in combination can help remove some kidney stones in susceptible individuals.

Magnesium stabilizes the internal structure of the cell and forms a bridge between proteins so as to stiffen cell membranes. It is also an essential co-factor in many intra-cellular enzymes and the body needs magnesium to build proteins themselves. Many hormones also depend upon magnesium in order to function.

4. Sodium and 5. Potassium

These are considered together because they are a natural pair of minerals that are closely interlinked (as are calcium and phosphorus).

Sodium and potassium are the body's two main positively charged ions and are found in solution all over the body. They are essential for maintaining the electrolyte balance of the body. Sodium chloride and potassium chloride (both tissue salts) are composed of positively charged metal parts (sodium or potassium) accompanied by equal numbers of negatively charged non-metal parts (chloride). Both potassium and sodium chloride are salty to taste and this is why most body fluids taste salty.

Sodium is found mainly outside the cells and potassium mainly inside. This difference in concentration produces an electrical potential across the cell membranes which is essential for nerve impulse transmission. The different concentrations of these salts also affects how cells react to any given electrical impulse.

All cells are permeable to potassium and sodium but a complex 'pump' mechanism keeps the balance just right across the cell membrane. If it weren't for the pump the concentrations of both ions would tend to equalize across cell membranes.

Perhaps the most vital role of sodium and potassium though lies in controlling the body's fluid balance. A delicately balanced mechanism exists to conserve sodium and potassium if intake is low and to excrete them via the urine if it is too high. Hormones control the excretion of these salts in such a way as to maintain body water (which makes up two thirds of our weight) at exactly the right levels.

If there is an excess of sodium in the body, water is retained, the body swells (oedema) and there is an increased risk of developing high blood pressure. Sodium depletion occurs much more rarely and is really seen only in conditions that promote profuse sweating (hot climates, working in boiler houses, or very high, prolonged fevers).

Sodium and potassium are also essential for nerve and muscle impulse transmission and have to be present in exactly the right proportions for this to occur. They thus have a role rather similar to calcium and magnesium—albeit in a lower concentration. An excess or deficiency of potassium, for example, has a positively bad effect on heart muscle and can cause even heart failure.

Lastly, sodium and potassium help control the acidity (pH) of the body's tissues in close association with proteins, bicarbonates and phosphates. These substances act as buffering agents to keep the acidity of the body just right under a wide variety of conditions.

6. Iron

This is the most important constituent of haemoglobin, the red blood pigment that carries oxygen. A lack of iron causes poor haemoglobin formation so that the body cannot get sufficient oxygen to its cells. This can produce tiredness, weakness and an inability to concentrate. Muscles tire easily too.

Muscles also contain an oxygen-binding, iron-containing pigment called myoglobin. This supplies an immediate source of oxygen during exercise.

Iron is also essential for the functioning of various enzymes called cytochromes. They are necessary for respiration inside cells where they are the final link in the oxygen supply chain that started in the lungs. Catalase is another oxygen-carrying enzyme present in cells and is necessary to detoxify hydrogen peroxide (a toxic cellular by-product).

Cellular iron is closely linked to disease resistance. Iron is essential for the adequate working of the immune system which is the body's main defence mechanism against invading micro-organisms. When the body iron levels are too low the bone marrow is unable to supply the necessary white blood cells to fight infection and resistance to disease is lowered. Anaemic people have a greater susceptibility to infections, especially those of the respiratory system, gastro-enteritis caused by a bacterium called *E. coli*, chronic infections of the teeth and gums and skin lesions such as boils and pimples.

In women the body sometimes gets short of iron because of heavy periods. Other conditions such as piles, gastric and duodenal ulcers, the long-term intake of aspirin, hiatus hernia, diverticulosis of the colon and excessive alcohol intake can also reduce the body's iron stores.

7. Fluoride

This trace element is present naturally in water supplies in certain areas of the country and is added to it in others.

Calcium fluoride improves dental development and strengthens bones by helping to deposit calcium. It reduces tooth decay in concentrations up to I part per million in drinking water. A deficiency of the mineral leads to poor bone and tooth formation and increased levels of dental caries (decay).

Fish eaten with the bones (tinned salmon and sardines, for example) and tea are excellent food sources. Too much of the mineral produces white mottling of the teeth but lower amounts reduce the amount of dental caries in children by up to 50 per cent. Our knowledge of fluoride in the body is still pretty poor but it is certainly essential in tiny amounts. There is considerable controversy over the fluoridation of water supplies, especially in the light of recent research which suggests there might be a link between fluoridation and cancer, birth defects and allergies.

8. Sulphate

This is present in the body as negatively charged ions in association with metallic ions (such as sodium, potassium, calcium, magnesium, etc.). Such mineral salts have many functions. Sodium sulphate is a very active diuretic (makes you pass more water than normal) because the kidney can't absorb the sulphate ions. Calcium sulphate is important in the production of white blood cells which are necessary for the defence of the body against foreign organisms. This salt is also effective in relieving abdominal pain and intestinal and gall bladder colic and is useful in treating diarrhoea.

Magnesium sulphate is used to treat magnesium deficiency states and is a component of many commonly used antacids.

9. Chloride

A negatively charged ion usually associated in the body with sodium and potassium to balance out their positive electrical charges. Chloride is not to be confused with chlorine, a highly poisonous gas. Chloride is usually obtained from dietary sources. Foods from animal sources such as meat, fish, poultry, milk and cheese are especially rich in it and seafoods tend to contain more than freshwater fish. It is almost always consumed as sodium chloride whether as table salt or in natural foods. Most fresh vegetables contain very little salt (sodium chloride) and most of this can be lost with prolonged cooking. Canned vegetables contain more salt than fresh or frozen ones. Unfortunately, many processed foods are rich in sodium chloride which can be hazardous if taken repeatedly over a long period.

Chloride levels in the body are usually related to sodium levels in the tissues. The toxic effects of sodium chloride are, however, all caused by the sodium and not the chloride, which has never been shown to be harmful in the body. Salt substitutes tend to be made of potassium chloride as the body seems to be able to handle potassium easily.

10 Silicon

This mineral is especially important for the normal production and repair of collagen (tough connective tissue or 'gristle') and bone. It is, therefore, essential for connecting bones and giving body structures strength and flexibility. It also helps to make the skin impermeable to liquids and maintains the elasticity of the walls of blood vessels, thus allowing them to constrict and dilate to vary the blood flow to any given area of the body.

These ten substances then are the basic constituents of the biochemic tissue salts but, as we have seen, the body needs many other minerals too. Everyone has heard of vitamins and accepts quite readily that they are essential for health. Very few on the other hand have really thought about the body's minerals and their importance. Minerals are, in reality, just as important as vitamins and, like vitamins, must be taken in food or as food supplements.

All of these minerals are inorganic—that is they are not living substances. Some are metals as we have seen (sodium, potassium, magnesium, calcium) and others non-metals (hydrogen, carbon, oxygen, phosphorus, etc.). A third group consists of the trace elements which are active and essential for life but which are only needed in the tiniest amounts. For example, the average adult needs about 800mg of calcium per day, which is 800,000 times his need for the trace element chromium.

The body's mineral levels are affected by the amount a person takes in his food; his age (many accumulate in the body with age); his sex; his family history; the presence of antagonistic substances in his food;

and the time of day the blood sample was taken. Different methods of estimation produce different results. Because there are so many variables and many of the minerals are present in such tiny amounts it can often be difficult to be certain about the actual dietary needs of any individual. Although dietary 'needs' have supposedly been calculated, there are substantial numbers of experts around the world who dispute that these are adequate. Excellent clinical results, for example, have been obtained in several conditions, using extremely high doses of vitamins—doses way above those recommended in nutrition manuals. Desirable levels of the major minerals are much less open to debate but the levels of the minor minerals (trace elements) are still disputed.

By and large minerals come ultimately from the soil (whether directly from plants or from animals which have fed on plants). Unfortunately, the quality of the soil around the world is falling as intensive farming leaches out the minerals. Certain valuable substances are replaced with nitrogenous fertilizers but this does not do anything to replenish the supplies of the trace elements that have been removed by repeating cropping. It has been known for years that goitre (a swollen thyroid gland) is caused by too little iodine in the soil of certain areas of the world (hence 'Derbyshire neck') and in some regions in Poland a greater incidence of cancer has been linked to a deficiency of magnesium in the soil. *Higher* than normal levels of certain minerals can accumulate as a result of pollution and this too can be harmful.

Sometimes the soil contains enough of an important trace element but not in a form which can be absorbed by the intestine. Cereals contain high concentrations of phytic acid which binds certain metals in food and makes them unavailable to the body. Other minerals are interdependent. Zinc absorption, for example, depends upon the presence of adequate amounts of phosphorus, iron and calcium.

Food processing does not destroy minerals but can make them unavailable to the body. The greatest loss of minerals occurs when refining foods. For example, 60 per cent of calcium is lost when refining flour, as is 71 per cent of the phosphorus, 90 per cent of the chromium, 85 per cent of the manganese and 88 per cent of the cobalt.

So, because of poor soil and the way we process, cook and store our foods, it is quite possible that many of us are short of certain minerals and trace elements and that diseases are the result. While the substances present in the tissue salts may possibly help to correct a deficiency, in my view we should be looking elsewhere for the main explanation as to how they work.

HOW DO BIOCHEMIC TISSUE SALTS WORK?

The short answer is that nobody knows but they probably work by virtue of their homoeopathic preparation method. So that we can understand more of how tissue salts work, let's look at the way homoeopathic medications are made.

When a homoeopath makes up a remedy he dilutes it with a solid (usually lactose) or a liquid (usually pure alcohol). If a solid is being used as the diluent then the remedy has to be ground up in a bowl to form an intimate mixture with the diluent. This grinding process is known as trituration. A fraction of the mixture is then taken and diluted tenfold (one part of the mixture added to nine parts of lactose) and this procedure repeated. The biochemic tissue salts are usually diluted 6 times in this way. This means that the original, active, salt is then present in a concentration of one part per million.

If the remedy is soluble, a similar procedure is followed but instead of grinding the remedy it is dissolved in the liquid by shaking vigorously. This is called succussion. The solutions thus produced are called 'potencies'.

The strength of the remedy is expressed as 1c, 2c, 3c, etc. as each successive hundredfold dilution and succussion is made. Because this method works in hundreds it is called centessimal as opposed to a parallel method of tenfold dilutions called decimal. In the UK this latter is expressed as 1x, 2x, 3x and on the continent of Europe as 1D, 2D, 3D. The tissue salts are usually supplied in potencies of 6x, as we have seen.

As the remedy is triturated or succussed time after time there comes a stage when there are very few molecules of the original remedy left in the solution. For example, by the time 12x is reached there may be only a tiny number of molecules of the remedy left in the solution, yet it would still be homoeopathically effective. The process by which a homoeopathic remedy becomes more and not less powerful as it is serially diluted and succussed is known as 'potentisation'. But why should tiny amounts of a remedy work at all? This is still a mystery and a major stumbling block between orthodox medicine and the homoeopathic world.

There are no easy explanations but a possible explanation lies in Avogadro's Hypothesis on matter which states that the number of molecules in one gram molecule of a substance is $6 \cdot 023 \times 10^{23}$. This means that theoretically if we dilute something to 10^{-24} (that is 1 and 24 '0's . . . i.e. 12x potency), there will be very few, if any, of the original molecules left. Recent work has shown, however, that the fluid in which they were originally dissolved might still carry information (in the form of energy) about the original substance. Put in another way, the original substance has 'imprinted' itself on to the fluid molecules. Knowledge of crystal structure and behaviour also indicates how a homoeopathic remedy associates with lactose to form new energy-rich lattices under the influence of physical grinding. Modern biochemists now happily discuss free energies being produced in biological reactions and a whole new area of science works on the assumption that energy rather than mass is at the heart of everything. By grinding or succussing an increasingly potent remedy with new diluent, more energy is built up in the molecules in rather the same way as people crammed into a railway compartment have more 'burst-out' energy when the train stops than a similar number of people sitting in a row of seats.

So the homoeopathic remedy is given to the patient in low concentration but in a high intrinsic energy state. It is this energy which is thought to be released to stimulate various bioenergetic systems in the body. It has also been suggested by nuclear physicists that such imprinted energy patterns have self-replicating qualities. This would help explain why homoeopathic remedies work so well—they may actually 'reproduce' in the bioenergetic systems of the body, unlike allopathic drugs that, as far as we know, are simply metabolized and excreted.

It may well be that some synthetic medicine molecules act in exactly similar ways to homoeopathic remedies in that many of them stimulate basic biochemical pathways at a cellular level. Drugs have a number of specific pharmacological effects which are desirable but often have other non-specific effects which are not wanted. It is rather like using a very long ladder to reach a window. Certainly the modern drug (long ladder) will get you to the window but the long overhang of the ladder above the top of the house may make the whole system unstable and potentially dangerous. Homoeopathic remedies are like short ladders that simply gain access to one desired window. Interestingly, many homoeopathic remedies act as specific 'short ladders' to many different windows though no one knows why or how they do so. Perhaps it is because they trigger basic body mechanisms that they do not need to be ultra-specific.

Perhaps then biochemic tissue salts, being potentised homoeopathically, act somehow to supercharge existing biochemical pathways involving the inorganic salts. At the moment no one can prove or disprove this theory but it seems a reasonable working hypothesis. To look at this another way let us see how modern scientific discoveries have enlarged our thinking about the absorption of a very commonly given mineral—iron.

It used to be thought that if you gave a person iron tablets to eat he would naturally and automatically absorb them all. Research has found that it is not quite this simple.

The absorption of minerals in the small intestine involves much more complex processes than was realized until recently. When iron is given as ferrous sulphate (the usual substance in iron tablets), the positively charged iron is attracted to the negatively charged intestinal wall and is eventually washed away by passing intestinal contents. The intestinal wall itself also reacts to get rid of the iron and most of it is lost. In addition to these hazards the iron may react with phytic acid (in cereals) and phosphate and tannic acid (from tea), all of which can render it insoluble and therefore useless to the body. Only about 3–10 per cent of dietary iron is absorbed, the rest is lost in the stools. If the body is short of iron though, its absorption is increased.

Some of the iron, however, is 'chelated' (coated with amino acids) by the body and because it is so protected, this iron is absorbed by the cells of the small intestine and soon finds its way into the blood which transports it around the body to perform its vital oxygen-carrying functions. This has led to the production of chelated iron (and other minerals) commercially.

Perhaps biochemic tissue salts have an activity akin to this process (but obviously not by coating the minerals with amino acids) in that they facilitate absorption in some as yet unproven way.

ARE THE TISSUE SALTS SAFE?

Undoubtedly the answer must be 'yes'. After a century's experience any dangerous side-effects would have been noticed. There has apparently been none. If they act by remedying defects in the body's normal but temporarily disordered mineral metabolism then there will be no ill-effects. If they are taken and the metabolic pathway does not need 'supercharging', they will simply be excreted. In any case, be careful to observe the manufacturer's recommended dosage.

There is one potential danger with the remedies but it is caused by the lactose and not by the active principles in the tablets. People who are sensitive to lactose should not take them or they will suffer the same symptoms they get when taking this milk sugar in milk (a bloated abdomen, cramping abdominal pains, nausea, loud tummy rumblings, watery diarrhoea, dehydration and vomiting). Although the tissue salt tablets are mainly sugar, the amount normally consumed should be of no concern to diabetics. If you are in any doubt, ask your doctor.

ARE THERE ANY SIDE-EFFECTS?

Apart from lactose intolerance, there are no known side-effects. Because the body has well-recognized ways of getting rid of all of the substances contained in the tissue salts and because they are given in such tiny amounts, there must be very little, if any, danger of overdose or side-effects. Were the same absolute amount as would be taken over many months to be taken in one dose, there could well be problems but this is completely contrary to the essence of tissue salt therapy as it is used in the UK.

HOW DO I CHOOSE WHICH ONE TO TAKE?

Over the last 100 years or so homoeopaths and others have found (by trial and error) which tissue salts seem to be helpful for which common ailments. These are listed alphabetically by symptoms on pages 41–52.

The salts are claimed to have the following useful actions:

1. *Calc. Fluor.* (Calcium Fluoride)—Deficient enamel of teeth.
2. *Calc. Phos.* (Calcium Phosphate)—Indigestion, teething problems, chilblains.
3. *Calc. Sulph.* (Calcium Sulphate)—Pimples during adolesence, skin slow to heal, sore lips.
4. *Ferr. Phos.* (Iron Phosphate)—Coughs, colds, chills, feverish chestiness. Take in alternation with *Kali. Mur.*
5. *Kali. Mur.* (Potassium Chloride)—Coughs, colds, wheeziness and

chestiness. Take in alternation with *Ferr. Phos.*

6. *Kali. Phos.* (Potassium Phosphate)—Temporary nerviness, nervous headache, or nervous indigestion due to worry or excitement.

7. *Kali. Sulph.* (Potassium Sulphate)—Minor skin eruptions with scaling or sticky exudation, brittle nails, catarrh.

8. *Mag. Phos.* (Magnesium Phosphate)—Cramp, flatulence, occasional minor pains.

9. *Nat. Mur.* (Sodium Chloride)—Watery colds with tears and runny nose, loss of smell or taste.

10. *Nat. Phos.* (Sodium Phosphate)—Indigestion, heartburn, 'rheumatic' pains.

11. *Nat. Sulph.* (Sodium Sulphate)—Queasiness, digestive upsets, aches and pains.

12. *Silica* (Silicon Dioxide)—Pimples or spots, brittle nails. Take in alternation with *Kali. Sulph.*

Combination 'A'
Ferr. Phos., Kali. Phos., mag. Phos.—Sciatica.

Combination 'B'
Calc. Phos., Kali. Phos., Ferr. Phos.—Edginess, convalescence.

Combination 'C'
Mag. Phos., Nat. Phos., Nat. Sulph., Silica—Acidity, heartburn, dyspepsia.

Combination 'D'
Kali. Mur., Kali. Sulph., Calc. Sulph., Silica—Minor skin ailments.

Combination 'E'
Calc. Phos., Mag. Phos., Nat. Phos., Nat. Sulph.—Flatulence, colicky pains, indigestion.

Combination 'F'
Kali. Phos., Mag. Phos., Nat. Mur., Silica—Nervous and migraine headache.

Combination 'G'
Calc. Fluor., Calc. Phos., Kali. Phos., Nat. Mur.—Backache, lumbago.

Combination 'H'
Mag. Phos., Kali. Sulph., Silica—Hay fever.

Combination 'I'
Ferr. Phos., Kali. Sulph., Mag. Phos.—Fibrositis, muscular pain.

Combination 'J'
Ferr. Phos., Kali. Sulph., Nat. Mur.—Coughs, colds, chestiness.

Combination 'K'
Kali. Sulph., Nat. Mur., Silica.—Brittle nails.

Combination 'L'
Calc. Fluor., Ferr. Phos., Nat. Mur.—Sedentary life-style.

Combination 'M'
Nat. Phos., Nat. Sulph., Kali. Mur., Calc. Phos.—Rheumatic pain.

Combination 'N'
Calc. Phos., Kali. Mur., Kali. Phos., Mag. Phos.—Menstrual pain.

Combination 'P'
Calc. Fluor., Calc. Phos., Kali. Phos., Mag. Phos.—Aching feet and legs.

Combination 'Q'
Ferr. Phos., Kali. Mur., Kali. Sulph., Nat. Mur.—Catarrh, sinus disorders.

Combination 'R'
Calc. Fluor., Calc. Phos., Ferr. Phos., Mag. Phos., Silica.—Infants' teething pains.

Combination 'S'
Kali. Mur., Nat. Phos., Nat. Sulph.—Stomach upsets, biliousness, sick headache.

The key to tissue salt medication is to isolate the symptom and to treat that. Schuessler claimed that the symptoms were a significant indication of which salt was needed.

In the treatment of certain acute (sudden onset) conditions different symptoms are apparent at different stages of the condition. In such cases the remedies should be changed and supplemented as the symptoms vary. For example, with the common cold a biochemic therapist would suggest *Ferr. Phos.* in the early stage together with *Kali. Mur.* to ease the stuffiness and congestion. As the watery discharge sets in *Nat. Mur.* would be prescribed instead. If the watery discharge became thick and containing mucus *Nat. Mur.* would be discontinued and *Calc. Sulph.* or *Kali. Sulph.* used instead.

If the choice of which salt to use is not apparent from the lists on pages 41–52, ask a homoeopath or a pharmacist who knows about them.

Medical men have for thousands of years claimed that illness is to some extent predetermined by the activity of the whole universe and for many hundreds of years astrological medicine was all the rage.

Today, few scientists and doctors have much time for this concept but modern research is beginning to make them think again. That there is a link between a person's astrological birth sign and his susceptibility to disease will, in my view, be proved within a decade or two and I am sure that astrological medicine will be legitimate within 30 years or so.

Quite simply, over the years the 12 tissue salts have been related to the 12 astrological star signs and it has been suggested that those born under any particular sign may be cured by 'their' tissue salt. The link that is proposed between each salt and its star sign is as follows:

Kali. Phos.	Aries
Nat. Sulph.	Taurus
Kali. Mur.	Gemini
Calc. Fluor.	Cancer
Mag. Phos.	Leo
Kali. Sulph	Virgo
Nat. Phos.	Libra
Calc. Sulph.	Scorpio
Silica	Sagittarius
Calc. Phos.	Capricorn
Nat. Mur.	Aquarius
Ferr. Phos.	Pisces

Some homoeopaths and other clinicians with a broad experience of the biochemic remedies claim that the best thing to do, if in doubt, is to take the tissue salt that complies with your star sign, alternating with the salt indicator for your particular symptom (see pages 41–52). If these two turn out to be the same remedy, take the 'opposite' star sign salt (the one 6 months apart from yours in the astrological calendar). This, it is claimed, is a good first-aid rule of thumb that can help pending a professional opinion from someone who has a more detailed knowledge of the remedies. It may even cure the complaint completely.

CAN THEY BE TAKEN WITH OTHER MEDICATIONS?

Experience shows that they can. Doctors and homoeopaths using these remedies have not found any reason to prevent them being taken if other (pharmaceutical or not) medications are also being used. Some homoeopaths even claim that the tissue salts are a useful background therapy on to which to add other active medications.

HOW DO I TAKE THEM?

Follow the instructions of your homoeopath or pharmacist or be guided by the instructions on the container. There really is no proven danger of overdose, so simply dissolve them on your tongue as directed. Because they dissolve instantaneously they enter the bloodstream at once through the tissues under the tongue.

HOW QUICKLY DO THEY ACT?

In acute (sudden onset, short-lived) conditions they seem to produce results in hours, especially if taken repeatedly in the early stages. In chronic (longstanding) conditions they can be taken for up to six months for the results to be apparent. Because of this profile of activity, tissue salts are particularly useful for short-lived, self-limiting conditions but they can, it is claimed, also be effective in certain chronic conditions. Dr Peter Gilbert, the London doctor with most experience of biochemic salts in the UK, maintains that because the turnover of minerals in the body is relatively slow it is inevitable that longstanding conditions caused by their deficiency will take weeks or months to improve simply because minerals already 'fixed' in the body's cells probably can't be influenced—they can only be replaced slowly with active, potentised minerals. Athough the tissue salts are distributed throughout the body and mix with the body's existing salts, there is a finite capacity for any one salt in the whole metabolic system. Because of this, potentised tissue salts to be effective may have to be taken for some time as they replace non-potentised salts in the body's total pool. This can take a particularly long time if the 'active' tissue salts are to affect long-term stores such as in teeth and bone, for example.

CAN THEY BE TAKEN ONLY AS TABLETS?

No—some of them can be used as external applications. For example cuts and abrasions can be rubbed with *Ferr. Phos.* after the injured part has been cleaned. Simply crush a few tablets and rub them in with clean fingers.

For lotions, dissolve 10 tablets in half a glass of water which has been previously boiled and left to cool. Dab the lotion on to the affected part. There are also preparations available containing certain of the tissue salts which can be used for minor skin ailments. One of these is claimed to be especially good for nappy rash.

WHEN SHOULD I CONSULT MY DOCTOR?

As we have seen, biochemic tissue salts are really only suitable as self-help remedies for minor, self-limiting ailments. They should not be used for more serious conditions unless they have been prescribed by a doctor who is familiar with their use.

In general if the condition for which you are taking the tissue salts is not getting better as you think it should, tell your doctor. Sometimes what seems like a simple and commonplace symptom can in fact be caused by something more serious, so don't persist with the salts, especially if the symptom is getting worse rather than improving. Ideally see a doctor or a medically qualified homoeopath to rule out other, more serious conditions before continuing with the treatment.

It is always best to play safe so, if in doubt, seek your doctor's opinion.

WHERE CAN I OBTAIN THE TISSUE SALTS?

There are two main sources of supply—health food shops and pharmacies. Some individual homoeopathic practitioners also make their own remedies.

Health food shops are the first port of call for most people because the vast majority of them sell biochemic tissue salts and can sometimes offer advice on how to use them. Increasing numbers of pharmacies are stocking them too. I see this as an exciting and important breakthrough because pharmacists are at least qualified to comment on common ailments and are currently used to helping people cope with everyday minor medical problems. They also know when to suggest a medical opinion. The National Pharmaceutical Association in the UK encourages their members to stock homoeopathic remedies and runs courses on them including biochemic remedies. Tissue salts are also available by mail from New Era Laboratories (the major manufacturer in the UK), 39 Wales Farm Road, London W3 6XH.

Up until the First World War, tissue salts were widely available from pharmacists, doctors and homoeopaths but the coming of powerful pharmaceutical preparations eclipsed them. Until 1952 herbal remedies were still in the pharmacopoeia (list of available medications) of pharmacists but were pushed out to make way for drugs whose effectiveness could be proven. There is no doubt that many a good baby was thrown out with the bath water as a result but there is equally no doubt that many of these simple natural remedies will find their place again. Indeed, many individual pharmacists are beginning to sell ginseng and other natural remedies and it can't be long before the giant chains follow suit.

CAN THEY BE USED FOR ANIMALS?

Homoeopathic remedies have been used for animals for over a century and biochemic tissue salts are no exception. Many people have found that their animals obtain similar benefits from the salts that they themselves do. Animals often respond very quickly to these remedies and, it is claimed, minor ailments can be cured just as in humans. Of course, as with treating humans, if things do not improve as you think they should, or things get worse, tell your vet.

Pet owners, vets and farmers have known for centuries that animals sometimes have bizarre appetites for strange 'foods'. A dog will eat grass, a pony the bark of a particular tree, and so on. Perhaps their instincts tell them that they need certain herbal remedies found in these things or perhaps the things they eat supply trace elements or other minerals in just the right dose to make them feel better. It will be years before we know the answers but the observation is an interesting one.

Talking of vets and farmers, it is a sobering thought that they, together with agricultural scientists, are probably more interested in and have more knowledge about inorganic salts and their importance than do doctors. Any good farmer will keep a careful eye on the mineral content of his soil and the intake of his animals. Increasing research has proven that some ailments in animals are caused by mineral and trace element deficiencies yet research in humans lags lamentably behind. Could it be that farmers value their highly-priced animals more than we value ourselves?

WHAT DO DOCTORS THINK OF THEM?

It is probably fair to say that the vast majority of doctors have never even heard of the tissue salts unless they are homoeopathically qualified so they cannot have formed an opinion about them. Homoeopaths (medically qualified or not) use them in varying degrees and they have been in the homoeopathic pharmacopoeia for over 100 years. There is increasing medical evidence that trace elements and other minerals are more important than the medical profession ever thought, and relatively new and as yet unavailable (to the public) measurement techniques such as hair analysis are linking particular diseases with the deficiency of certain minerals and trace elements. As these become better recognized and more acceptable to the medical world generally, there is little doubt that the biochemic remedies will be looked at more closely. After all, doctors used them at the end of the last century and the beginning of this so perhaps the medical profession will come back to them. It is well known that the medical world tends to accept only things that can be *proven* to be valuable. Since the discovery of the vitamins there has been little debate that they are valuable and even vital to health but physicians even as recently as the start of this century were still talking solely about the energy value of food. Since then the scientific and medical worlds have been content to add 'essential' substances to their list of what is thought necessary for life. Unfortunately, current knowledge is just as patchy and unsatisfactory as it was before the discovery of the vitamins—it is just as deficient in other ways, as yet unrecognized by medicine.

Unfortunately, there have been no clinical trials done on tissue salts and this is a black mark from the orthodox medical point of view. Dr Peter Gilbert who, as we have seen, was something of an early pioneer with his father in this field, did some simple clinical trials when he and his father, Dr Henry Gilbert, ran the Biochemic School in London. Because the medical press of the day refused to publish the results they have been lost to posterity but he and his father were convinced of the effectiveness of the salts—and so were his patients. Dr Gilbert claims an 80 per cent success rate in most of the conditions he sees although sometimes he finds it necessary to use acupuncture along with the tissue salts. However, the orthodox medical profession is unlikely to accept them as more than just a safe placebo except after carefully controlled, double-blind trials to prove that they do in fact work. We can prove so little about the tissue salts in satisfactory scientific terms and about the subtle substances in our food generally that we are bound to be fumbling around for decades to come. In the meantime millions of people will continue to take the tissue salts and to get relief from them, whatever the explanation of their efficacy.

WHAT ARE THEY USED FOR?

By and large it is fair to say that the biochemic tissue salts are best used for minor everyday aches, pains and ailments. They are not intended to be used *instead* of medical treatment prescribed by your doctor. They can, however, be used *as well as* prescribed medications because experience has shown that this is completely safe.

If you are ill you will have to make a decision as to whether you want to see your doctor straight away or whether you will try to cure yourself. I say 'cure yourself' but in reality it is your body that heals itself. As we have already seen, about 8 out of 10 of all those going to their doctors have self-limiting conditions, so the chances are that what you have may well correct itself given time and a healthy body.

Unfortunately, we have all become impatient in today's rush-along world and want results rather more quickly than the body can deliver them. This unnatural haste to get better takes people to their doctors in droves for remedies for conditions that would anyway have got better.

The biochemic tissue salts are safe, self-help remedies that can fill the waiting gap while your body heals itself *but* unlike drugs form your doctor the tissue salts will do you no harm and may even trigger the body's natural healing processes in some, as yet unknown, way.

There are literally thousands of minor ailments that any one of us can suffer from, so what I have done is to group some of the commoner ones together under alphabetical headings for ease of reference. Obviously, there comes a time when any given symptom or complaint *must* be reported to a doctor if it has not improved or disappeared completely. I have put the number of days beyond which it could be dangerous to delay seeking medical help in brackets after each entry. The number tells you the maximum number of days you should continue with home remedies such as the tissue salts before going for medical help. If there is no number, simply be guided by common sense as usual and see your doctor if you are at all worried.

Finally, I cannot personally guarantee the success of the tissue salts in the conditions I've listed. The remedies for these conditions have been arrived at over more than a century by trial and error by practitioners— many of them homoeopaths and medical doctors.

If ever you are worried about any symptom, especially if it persists, always consult your doctor or a medically qualified homoeopath.

PART THREE

SELECTING
A REMEDY

SOME COMMON AILMENTS AND THE TISSUE SALTS CLAIMED TO BE OF HELP

(Based on the observations of Dr Schuessler and others)

Always continue to take prescribed medicines as usual—add tissue salts if appropriate

A

Abdomen, bloated: *Kali. Sulph.*, *Mag. Phos.* (2)
Acid regurgitation: *Nat Phos.*
Acne: *Calc. Sulph.*
Anaemia: *Ferr. Phos.*, *Calc. Phos.*
Anus—itching of: *Nat Phos.*, *Calc. Fluor.*(10)
      —cracks and fissures of: *Calc. Fluor.*
Anxiety: *Kali. Phos.*
Asthma: *Kali. Phos.*, *Mag. Phos.*

B

Beard area, pimples: *Calc. sulph.*
Bed-wetting in children: *Kali. Phos.*, *Nat. Phos.*, *Ferr. Phos.*, *Nat. Mur.*, *Calc. Phos.* (28)
Belching—with taste of food: *Ferr. Phos.*
      —with sour taste: *Nat. Phos.*
Blisters: *Nat. Mur.*

—with thick, white contents: *Kali. Mur.*
Blockage of tear ducts from cold weather: *Nat. Mur.*
Bloodshot eyes: *Ferr. Phos.* (2)
Bronchitis: *Ferr. Phos.* (28)
Burns: *Kali. Mur.*
    —suppurating: *Calc. Sulph.*

C

Callosities: *Calc. Fluor.*
Catarrh in ear, causing mild deafness: *Kali. Sulph., Kali. Mur.* (7)
Chapped hands from cold: *Calc. Fluor.*
Chapping of lips: *Calc. Fluor.*
Chilblains on hands and feet: *Calc. Phos., Kali. Phos., Kali. Mur.*
Chilliness, especially in the back, watery saliva, heavy headache: *Nat Mur.*
Circulation poor: *Kali. Phos., Calc. Phos., Calc. Fluor.*
Colds—early stages: *Ferr. Phos.*
Colic in infants: *Mag. Phos.* (1)
Constant desire to open bowels: *Kali. Mur.* (7)
Constipation with light-coloured stools: *Kali. Mur.*
Cough—acute, painful, short and irritating: *Ferr. Phos.*
    —better in cool air: *Kali. Sulph.*
    —convulsive bouts: *Mag. Phos.*
    —hard, dry: *Ferr. Phos.* (7)
    —irritating, painful: *Ferr. Phos.* (7)
    —loud and noisy: *Kali. Mur.*
    —spasmodic: *Mag. Phos.*
    —worse in evening: *Kali. Sulph.*
    —worse lying down: *Mag. Phos.*
    —worse in warm room: *Kali. Sulph.*
Coughing to clear throat: *Calc. Phos.*
Cracking of joints: *Nat. Phos.*
Cracking noises in ear—on blowing nose: *Kali. Mur.*
               —on swallowing: *Kali. Mur.*
Cracks in palms of hands: *Calc. Fluor.*
Craving for salt or salty food: *Nat. Mur.*
Cries easily: *Kali. Phos.* (28)

Cystitis: *Kali. Mur., Ferr. Phos., Kali. Phos., Mag. Phos.* (7)

D

Dandruff: *Nat. Mur., Kali. Sulph.*
Depression: *Kali. Phos., Calc. Phos., Nat. Mur.* (28)
Despondency: *Kali. Phos.*
Diarrhoea—after eating greasy, fatty food: *Kali. Mur.*
     —alternating with constipation: *Nat. Mur.* (7)
     —with green, sour-smelling stools: *Nat. Phos.*
     —like water: *Nat. Mur.* (3)
     —with greenish stools or vomiting of bile: *Nat. Sulph.* (2)
     —with clay-coloured, slimy stools and swelling of the abdomen:
        Kali. Mur. (7)
     —with yellow, slimy, purulent matter: *Kali. Sulph.* (3)
Discharge—from ear, thick and white: *Kali. Mur.*
     —from eye—golden-yellow, creamy: *Nat. Phos.* (3)
     —from eye—thick, white mucus: *Kali. Mur.* (3)
     —from eye—thick, yellow: *Calc. Sulph.* (3)
     —from eye—greenish, serous: *Kali. Sulph.* (3)
Dizziness from exhaustion: *Kali. Phos.*
Drooping of eyelids: *Kali. Phos., Mag. Phos.* (7)
Drowsiness in the elderly: *Silica*
Dryness of nose, with scabbing: *Nat. Mur., Silica*

E

Earache—with beating, throbbing pain: *Ferr. Phos.* (1)
     —with swelling of lymph nodes (glands) or tonsils: *Kali. Mur.* (3)
     —with yellow discharge: *Kali. Sulph.* (2)

F

Face—coldness or numbness of: *Calc. Phos.* (10)
    —flushed, cold sensation at nape of neck: *Ferr. Phos.*
    —neuralgia with tears: *Nat. Mur.* (10)
    —neuralgia with shifting pains: *Kali. Sulph.* (10)
    —neuralgia with shooting pains: *Mag. Phos.* (10)

—neuralgia with spasmodic pain: *Mag. Phos.* (10)
—neuralgia aggravated by cold: *Mag. Phos.* (10)
—neuralgia relieved by hot applications: *Mag. Phos.*
Fainting—tendency to: *Kali. Phos.*
Fatty food disagrees: *Kali. Mur., Nat. Phos.* (28)
Feet twitch during sleep: *Nat. Sulph.*
Fever—with chills and cramps: *Mag. Phos., Ferr. Phos.*
   —first stages of: *Ferr. Phos.*
Flatulence—with distress about heart: *Kali. Phos., Nat. Phos.* (14)
         —with pains in left side: *Kali. Phos.*
Flatulent colic: *Nat. Phos., Nat. Sulph., Mag. Phos.*
Flatulent colic with green sour-smelling stools: *Nat. Phos.*
Frequent passing of urine, sometimes scalding: *Kali. Phos.* (3)

G

Gastric symptoms—aggravated by acid drinks: *Mag. Phos.* (28)
             —aggravated by cold drinks: *Calc. Phos., Mag. Phos.*
             —relieved by cold drinks: *Ferr. Phos.*
Gout: *Nat. Phos., Nat. Sulph., Ferr. Phos.*
Gum-boil: *Silica* (2)
       —before pus begins to form: *Kali. Mur.*
Gums—bleed easily: *Kali. Phos.* (7)
   —pale: *Calc. Phos.*
   —hot, swollen and inflamed: *Ferr. Phos.* (5)
   —swollen: *Kali. Mur.* (5)

H

Hair loss: *Kali. Sulph., Silica, Nat. Mur.* (28)
Halitosis (bad breath): *Kali Phos.*
Hands—involuntary motions of: *Mag. Phos.*
     —twitch during sleep: *Nat. Sulph.*
Hard to wake in morning: *Calc. Phos.*
Hay fever: *Mag. Phos., Nat. Mur., Silica*
Head—involuntary shaking of: *Mag. Phos.*
Headache—at crown of head: *Nat. Phos.*
       —from mental work: *Kali. Phos.*

—nervous: *Kali. Phos.*
—on waking: *Nat. Phos.*
—relieved by cool air: *Kali. Sulph.*
—relieved by relaxation: *Kali. Phos.*
—with biliousness, bitter taste: *Nat. Sulph.*
—with drowsiness: *Nat. Mur.* (1)
—with neuralgia: *Kali. Phos., Mag. Phos.*
—with neuralgia and humming in the ears. *Kali. Phos.*
—with pain over eye: *Ferr. Phos.* (3)
—with pain in temples: *Ferr. Phos., Nat. Phos.*
—with sadness: *Kali. Phos.* (28)
—with sharp, shooting pains: *Mag. Phos.* (3)
—with throbbing pain: *Ferr. Phos.*
—with unrefreshing sleep: *Nat. Mur.*
—with vomiting of acid or sour fluids: *Nat. Phos.* (1)
—with vomiting of bile: *Nat. Sulph.* (1)
—with vomiting of undigested food: *Ferr. Phos.* (1)
Heartburn: *Calc. Phos., Nat. Sulph., Silica* (28)
Herpetic eruptions on skin: *Nat. Mur.* (3)
Hiccough: *Mag. Phos.* (2)
Hoarseness: *Calc. Phos.* (7)
Hopelessness: *Nat. Mur.* (7)

I

Impatience and nervousness: *Kali. Phos.*
Incontinence—from nervous debility: *Kali. Phos.*
            —from weakness of sphincter: *Ferr. Phos.*
            —while walking or coughing: *Nat. Mur.* (28)
Indigestion—with griping pains: *Mag. Phos.*
            —with watery fluid or sour taste in the mouth: *Nat. Mur.*
            —with watery vomiting and salty taste in the mouth: *Nat. Mur.* (2)
Inflammation—first stage: *Ferr. Phos.*
            —second stage: *Kali. Mur.*
Irritability: *Kali. Phos.*
Itching of skin: *Kali. Phos., Calc. Phos.*

J

Jerking of limbs during sleep: *Silica, Nat. Sulph.*

L

Laryngitis: *Calc. Phos., Ferr. Phos.* (5)
Lips—cracked: *Calc. Fluor.*
   —twitching: *Mag. Phos.* (5)
Loose morning stools, worse in cold, wet weather: *Nat. Sulph.*
Looseness of bowels—in old people: *Nat. Sulph.*
         —with watery stools. *Nat. Sulph.*
Lumbago: *Calc. Phos., Ferr. Phos., Nat. Phos.*
      —from strains: *Calc. Fluor.*
Lump in throat on swallowing: *Nat. Sulph.* (7)
Lymph nodes (glands) around the ear swollen; snapping and cracking noises
   in the ear: *Kali. Mur.* (2)

M

Memory poor: *Calc. Phos., Kali. Phos., Mag. Phos.*
Menopausal symptoms—hot flushes: *Ferr. Phos.*
   alternating with *Kali. Sulph.*
            —nervousness; depression, irritability, anxiety: *Kali. Phos.* (28)
            —weakness, feeling run down: *Calc. Phos.*
Migraine: *Kali. Phos., Nat. Sulph.* (7)
Morning sickness: *Ferr. Phos.*
         —with frothy, watery phlegm: *Nat. Mur.*
         —with vomiting of sour mucus and acid taste in mouth:
            Nat. Phos.
         —with bilious vomiting: *Nat. Sulph.*

N

Nails brittle: *Silica, Kali. Sulph., Calc. Fluor.*
Nasal catarrh—with fever: *Ferr. Phos.*
         —with stuffiness: *Kali. Mur.*
         —worse in evening: *Kali. Sulph.*

Nasal discharge—albuminous: *Calc. Phos.*
    —clear watery: *Nat. Mur.*
    —lumpy, yellow: *Calc. Fluor.*
    —purulent, bloody: *Calc. Sulph.*
    —slimy, yellow or greenish: *Kali. Sulph.*
    —thick, white: *Kali. Mur.*
    —yellow, creamy: *Nat. Phos.*
    —yellow, offensive: *Calc. Fluor.*
Nasal polypi: *Calc. Phos.* (28)
Neck lymph nodes (glands) painful and aching: *Calc. Phos.* (3)
Neck muscles stiff: *Ferr. Phos.*
Nettlerash: *Calc. Phos.*
   —after becoming overheated: *Nat. Mur.*
Neuralgia—at night: *Calc. Phos.*
   —periodic: *Mag. Phos., Nat. Mur.*
   —relieved by gentle motion: *Kali. Phos.*
   —relieved by gentle relaxation. *Kali. Phos.*
   —with depression: *Kali. Phos.* (28)
   —with excess saliva: *Nat Mur.*
   —with flow of tears: *Nat. Mur.*
   —with shifting pains: *Kali. Sulph.*
   —with weakness: *Kali. Phos.*
   —worse in cold weather: *Nat. Mur.*
   —worse in the morning: *Nat. Mur.*
Neuralgic pain in the eyes with tears: *Nat. Mur.* (7)
Nose bleed: *Ferr. Phos.* (1)
Nostrils—inflammation at edges: *Silica*

P

Periods—ceased in non-menopausal women with depression, lassitude, debility, headaches and irritability: *Kali. Phos.*
   —ceased in non-menopausal women with 'full' feeling in abdomen: *Kali. Sulph.*
   —heavy, too frequent and too profuse: *Ferr. Phos.*
   —heavy, with bearing-down pains: *Calc. Fluor.*
   —painful, relieved by heat: *Mag. Phos.*

—painful, with vomiting, bright red flow, flushed face: *Ferr. Phos.*, alternate with *Mag. Phos.* during attack.

—painful, in pale, tearful, sensitive woman: *Kali. Phos.* alternate with *Ferr. Phos.* (2 cycles)

—scanty in young girls: *Nat. Mur.*

Perspiration—excessive: *Calc. Phos., Kali. Phos.*

　　　　　—lack of: *Kali. Sulph.*

　　　　　—sour smelling: *Nat. Phos., Silica*

　　　　　—to promote: *Kali. Sulph.*

Pharyngitis: *Calc. Phos.*

Pharynx, dryness and rawness of: *Nat. Mur.*

Phlegm—albuminous: *Calc. Phos.*

　　　　—salty: *Nat. Mur.*

　　　　—slips back: *Kali. Sulph.*

　　　　—thick, yellow or green: *Silica* (5)

　　　　—tiny yellow lumps: *Calc. Fluor.* (5)

　　　　—watery: *Nat. Mur.*

　　　　—yellow or green, slimy: *Kali. Sulph.* (5)

Pimples—on face: *Calc. Sulph.*

　　　　—with itching: *Calc. Phos.*

Pregnancy: *Kali. Phos.* and *Calc. Phos.* from 3-6 months before birth

Pustules on face: *Silica, Kali. Mur.*

R

Rattling in chest: *Kali. Mur., Nat. Mur.* (7)

Retention of stools: *Nat. Mur.*

Rheumatism: *Ferr. Phos., Nat. Phos., Nat. Sulph., Silica*

　　　　　—with swelling: *Kali. Mur.*

S

Saliva, excess of: *Nat. Mur.* (28)

Salivary glands inflamed with excessive amounts of saliva: *Nat. Mur.* (5)

Scabs on skin: *Nat. Sulph.*

　　　　　　—yellow: *Calc. Sulph.*

Sciatica: *Mag. Phos., Ferr. Phos.*

Sensitiveness: *Kali. Phos.*

Shingles: *Kali. Mur., Nat. Mur.*
    —for the pain: *Ferr. Phos. (powder applied locally), Mag. Phos.* (7)
Shivering at beginning of fever: *Calc. Phos., Ferr. Phos.*
Shyness: *Kali. Phos.*
Sick headache from gastric upset: *Nat. Sulph.*
Skin—dry: *Calc. Fluor., Kali. Sulph.*
    —dry, hot and burning, lack of perspiration: *Kali. Sulph.*
    —festers easily: *Calc. Sulph.*
    —greasy scales: *Kali. Phos.*
    —heals slowly and suppurates easily after injuries: *Silica*
    —scaling of: *Calc. Phos., Kali. Sulph.*
    —to encourage the formation of new skin: *Kali. Sulph.*
    —withered and wrinkled: *Kali. Phos.*
Sleep, unrefreshing: *Nat. Mur.*
Sleepiness: *Nat. Mur.*
    —in morning: *Nat. Mur.*
Sleeplessness from nervous causes: *Kali. Phos.* (28)
Smell, loss or perversion of, not connected with a cold: *Mag. Phos.* (28)
Smell, loss of, with dryness and rawness of the pharynx
Sneezing: *Silica, Nat. Mur.*
Soreness of mouth: *Kali. Mur.* (7)
Spasmodic twitching of eyelids: *Mag. Phos.*
Sprains: *Ferr. Phos.*
Stings of insects: *Nat. Mur.* (applied locally)
Stomach feels bloated: *Calc. Phos.*
Stools dry and often produce fissures at the anus: *Nat. Mur.*
Strains: *Ferr. Phos.*
Stuffy cold with yellow, lumpy mucus: *Calc. Fluor.*
    —with greenish mucus: *Kali. Sulph., Silica*
Stye: *Silica*
Sulphurous odour of gas from bowels: *Kali. Sulph.*
Suppuration of throat: *Calc. Sulph.*
Sweating at night: *Nat. Mur., Silica., Calc. Phos.*

T

Taste in mouth—acid or sour: *Nat. Phos.*

   —bitter: *Nat. Sulph.*

   —unpleasant: *Nat. Sulph., Kali. Phos.*

   —unpleasant in morning: *Calc. Phos.*

Tears—when going into the cold air: *Nat. Mur.*

  —with neuralgia in the eyes: *Nat. Mur., Mag. Phos.*

Teeth—loose: *Calc. Fluor.* (28)

  —sensitive to cold: *Mag. Phos.*

  —sensitive to touch: *Mag. Phos., Calc. Fluor.*

Teething—with drooling: *Nat. Mur.*

   —late: *Calc. Phos.*

Thirst: *Nat. Mur.*

  —with excessive amount of watery urine: *Nat. Mur.* (14)

Throat—constricted feeling in: *Mag. Phos.* (7)

  —dry, red and inflamed: *Ferr. Phos.*

  —raw feeling, without inflammation: *Nat. Phos.*

  —sore: *Ferr. Phos.*

  —sore and dry: *Nat. Mur.*

  —sore in singers and speakers: *Ferr. Phos.*

  —sore when swallowing, with tender neck: *Silica* (3)

  —tickling in: *Calc. Fluor.*

Throat ulcers—with thick yellow discharge: *Silica*

   —with white or grey patches: *Kali. Mur.*

Thrush in mouth: *Kali. Mur.* (3)

Tiredness from overwork: *Kali. Phos.*

Tongue—blisters on tip: *Nat. Mur., Calc. Phos.*

  —cracked: *Calc. Fluor.*

  —chronic swelling of: *Calc. Fluor.* (14)

  —coated, brownish: *Kali. Phos.*

  —coated, creamy on back part: *Nat. Phos.*

  —coated, dirty, greenish-grey, with bitter taste: *Nat. Sulph.*

  —coated, greyish-white: *Kali. Mur.*

  —coated, yellow and slimy: *Kali. Sulph.*

  —coated, yellow on back part: *Nat. Phos.*

  —dark red and inflamed: *Ferr. Phos.* (14)

  —numb: *Calc. Phos.* (3)

  —pimples on tip of: *Calc. Phos.*

  —swollen: *Kali. Mur., Calc. Phos.* (3)

—ulcers on: *Silica*
Tonsillitis, after pus has begun to form: *Silica*
Tonsils—chronic enlargement of: *Calc. Phos.*
    —grey-white patches on: *Kali. Mur.*
    —inflamed: *Ferr. Phos.*
Tooth decay (dental caries): *Calc. Fluor., Calc. Phos.* (7)
Tooth enamel—brittle: *Calc. Fluor.*
      —rough and thin: *Calc. Fluor.*
Toothache—aggravated by hot liquids: *Ferr. Phos.*
    —relieved by cold applications: *Ferr. Phos.*
    —relieved by hot applications: *Mag. Phos.*
    —with excessive flow of saliva or tears: *Nat. Mur.*
    —with neuralgia of face: *Mag. Phos.* (3)
    —with swelling of gums or cheeks: *Kali. Mur., Ferr. Phos.* (3)
Travel sickness: *Kali. Phos., Nat. Phos.*
Trembling hands: *Mag. Phos.*
Trembling and involuntary motion of the hands: *Mag. Phos.* (7)
Trembling and involuntary shaking of the head: *Mag. Phos.* (7)

U

Ulcers—at corners of mouth: *Silica*
    —in mouth, grey: *Kali. Phos.*
    —in mouth, white: *Kali. Mur.*
Upper respiratory tract inflammation in the early stages: *Ferr. Phos.*
Urinary retention (spasmodic): *Mag. Phos.*

V

Vaginal discharge—white, non-irritating: *Kali. Mur.*
    —scalding, yellow or orange: *Kali. Phos.* (3)
    —yellow or greenish, slimy or watery: *Kali. Sulph.* (3)
Varicose veins and ulceration: *Calc. Fluor.*
Vomiting—after cold drinks: *Calc. Phos.* (2)
    —bile: *Nat. Sulph.* (3)
    —sour, acid fluids: *Nat. Phos.* (2)
    —thick, white phlegm: *Kali. Mur.* (2)
    —undigested food: *Ferr. Phos.* (2)

W

Warts: *Kali. Mur.*
    —on palms of hand. *Nat. Mur.*
Waterbrash: *Nat. Mur.*
Weeps easily: *Nat. Mur.*
Wounds discharging pus: *Calc. Sulph.*

Y

Yellow, sallow or jaundiced face: *Nat. Sulph.* (3)

DO PEOPLE ACTUALLY USE THEM?

Yes, they certainly do. Sales of the tissue salts and especially of the combinations are rocketing. To a certain extent this simply reflects the increasing public interest in natural cures and health foods generally. Over the last few years, health food sales have increased greatly and, at a time when small shops are closing everywhere, new health food shops are springing up. The health food trade looks set for a further boom as large supermarket chains start to stock health products. There is little doubt that if the tissue salts were more widely available through chemists' shops and supermarkets they would sell in even larger amounts. What used to be considered a 'specialist', 'cranky', middle class market has blossomed to embrace all age groups, all social classes and all kinds of very normal and ordinary people. Big business has recognized this and 'natural' products abound throughout the food, cosmetics, toiletries and health areas.

The growth in use of tissue salts is a part of this movement but is also something more because in addition to being 'natural' they are seen to be harmless yet effective for a host of minor, everyday ailments.

As there is no better available evidence of their efficacy than that from convinced and satisfied patients, here are a few selected quotations. Obviously they are self-selected because those who wrote the letters obtained benefits and were sufficiently motivated to write to the company that makes the salts they used. However, nationwide and international sales of tissue salts suggests that these letters are not at all unusual. After all, people would not continue to use them if they did not work. Undoubtedly many people will get no relief with the tissue salts but this can equally well be said for various pharmaceutical preparations with proven potency and effectiveness which cost a great deal more.

SOME QUOTATIONS FROM SATISFIED PATIENTS

'I would like to thank you for the New Era Biochemic Tissue Salts which I have used, on occasions, for several years now. I am especially grateful for "Combination R" which has acted faster than any painkiller in curing wisdom-teething pains! I have been taking 4 tablets every 15–30 minutes and the pain usually disappears after either the first or second dose. After several months still only half a tooth is showing and it appears that the whole process will take a while yet, so my supplies have not outlived their usefulness. I also have to take Combination K every day, otherwise my nails keep breaking.

Once again, thank you for making these Biochemic Tissue Salts available.'

Miss E.G., Oxford

'I find the tissue salts very effective indeed—I take them regularly and when I get a particularly acute attack of stiffness, they act quite quickly, taken every half-hour, as suggested. I have a certain amount of osteoarthritis and have had a hip replacement—which settled that problem but created others, as operations are apt to do, and I'm often extremely stiff particularly below and around where the muscle was cut, and round my lumbar region. When this happens I find that the tablets help a great deal. Of course, I do other things as well—keep exercising, keep off unsuitable foods and drinks, sugar, etc. and I eat plenty of fresh, raw vegetables.'

Mrs M.G.R., Glos.

'I have suffered from premenstrual headaches which are really bad and even my husband says I look awful during them. My doctor gave me tablets which didn't help and I also have severe anaemia. I read in a paper about Nervone (a tissue salt nerve nutrient)—and as a last resort tried it. I have had it now for a year and I very seldom have a headache—if I do it's very mild.'

Mrs R., Middlesex

'Having taken a combination of tissue salts for over twenty years with great relief I have been unable to obtain them for months. This week I managed to buy the last bottle from the chemist. My legs had been very painful and I was naturally pleased. I can truthfully say that within two days I am feeling much better. As I am a widowed senior citizen and on a widow's pension as my only income, is it possible for you to supply me with a large pack as it is a great saving to me.'

Mrs F.M., Bath

'From the age of 14 I have suffered from dandruff and falling hair. I was introduced to the tissue salts and found my symptoms described under *Kali. Sulph.* I found a great improvement after the first day of treatment. I have very little dandruff, my hair is not falling out as much as it was and the itchy discomfort on the scalp soon goes when the tablets are taken and returns within hours if the treatment is stopped. I take 4 three or four times a day. I have tried Combination K but without success. My wife finds a great improvement in her state of mind after taking *Kali. Phos.*

My step-father has always suffered with catarrh and a rash on his forehead. Both these complaints are cleared with regular use of the tissue salts. A colleague at work had suffered with piles for 10 or 12 years causing great discomfort. His doctor had given him everything there was to relieve the irritation and pain but if anything did work at all the remedy was as unpleasant as the condition. He was a great sceptic of my esoteric knowledge but, when he had overheard a conversation, asked if there was anything on haemorrhoids. I gave him the book to ascertain which salt he required. He told me weeks after that, since taking the tablets, he had not felt any more discomfort at all.'

Mr P.C., Lincoln

'I purchased some of your tissue salts ('Q' for catarrh and sinus disorders) perhaps two months ago. As I don't usually take medicines, when I do I normally take smaller doses than quoted because they can have a strong effect on me. In this case I didn't take them immediately but, one morning when my nose and throat were troublesome with catarrh, I took 2 tablets (the child's dose) and forgot about it.

It was about three hours later that I suddenly realized I could breathe freely and didn't have mucus coming into my mouth as was my normal routine every morning for a few hours (and through the daytime). Since then I have taken them continually, sometimes 2 in the morning, occasionally 2 in the evening, if necessary. I feel very free of catarrh and am most grateful and very surprised.'

Miss B.J., Kent

'I am writing to say thank you for the combination salt tablets you make. I did not know where to put my legs, I had so much pain in them. I have tried everything and a very old lady told me about your tablets. I got some next day and have been on them only two weeks. I can't say thank you enough. I have had great relief and I will recommend them to all my friends who have the same trouble as I have had. I will never be without a box in my home. What a change to be able to get up from the chair, with a spring, as I am now able to do and come home from shopping 'legs alright'. I had to write and tell you, I am so pleased and thank God I met that lady.'

Mrs F., Accrington

'I am writing to tell you how effective I have found some of your tissue salts in the treatment of certain disorders. For instance just recently *Calc. Fluor.* has begun to put my teeth in order. Until recently I had two sensitive biting surfaces and was unable to chew food on my right jaw but now it is quite normal. The dentist was unable to find anything wrong.'

Mrs H., Wiltshire

'I have a layman's interest in homoeopathy and have recently switched to using your Combination M for osteoarthritis for the past three weeks. I can only say that the results are good.'

Mrs B., South Africa

'I am 78 years of age and had a stroke five years ago which affected my left arm and leg. On the doctor's instructions I dieted and lost weight and since have been a vegetarian except for eggs, milk and fish. I recovered movements, but my walking was bad and uneven.

About three years ago I took New Era G and became much better and now I am quite active and healthy for my age. I keep a large garden in order and walk moderate distances, though I get tired. I am grateful to

Dr Schuessler for his research and remedies.'

Miss H., Isle of Wight

'I just had to tell you your combination tablets are wonderful. I have been in England on holiday and while there my legs were aching. I bought a box of your tablets in Liverpool and they are wonderful, only we can't get them here.'

Mrs C., Australia

'I have recently found relief from Combination C tablets for heartburn which were passed on to me by a friend. I am wondering if your company has any preparations which help hot flushes?'

Mrs B., Bristol

'I am writing to say how much benefit I have received from your Biochemic Tissue Salts.

For the past year or so I have taken the Combination Salts for coughs, colds, etc.; also for nervous disability but find on taking the individual *Ferr. Phos.* I have had tremendous relief, especially as I have been subject to very throaty, chesty colds more than usual. I take them frequently when I am like this. I would like to ask if I am able to take them often and always, only I don't want to get so used to them and then find that they may not help me as much. I really must say that to me they are like a life-saver when I feel so poorly with these colds.'

Miss W., Bristol

'I have reason to be very grateful to you for putting on the market your wonderful tissue salts. A few months ago I developed a very bad throat. The doctor just could not understand what could be wrong. I had tried just about everything and was getting very worried as it was getting worse. Then by chance I saw a book about the salts in a health food shop. After reading it and getting the information I needed I tried your tissue salt *Ferr. Phos.* Within half an hour I began to feel better and I have not looked back since. Thank you again for your wonderful product.'

Miss P.A.N., Lincolnshire

'Just a note to thank you for the relief I have got from chilblains. After taking the tablets for two days all the wounds on my hands were healed up.'

Mrs McM., Eire

'I have recently commenced using your tablets (Combination F) in an attempt to reduce the incidence of migraine. I have to date found the tablets apparently effective in that I have been virtually free of migraine for one month whereas I could normally have expected a couple of attacks a week.'

Mr J.R.C., Surrey

'I found the tissue salts very effective after only one day. Everything I ate was giving me indigestion: my stomach was like a hard football. The more I ate the worse I became. I have been like this for years. I now feel like a new woman after taking Combination E for flatulence, colic and indigestion. Words cannot express my gratitude. Thank you very much.'

Mrs V.S., N. Ireland

I have been using Schuessler salts for over 20 years and find the following particularly useful. I have not stuck to any long-term treatment for any length of time but these remedies taken promptly have, I am sure, prevented the development of many irksome minor ailments.

My experiences are as follows:

Calc. Fluor.—Two or three half-hourly doses will normally clear dragging pains or period pains in the lower back.

Calc. Sulph.—Two or three half-hourly doses taken at the very first indication of a cold (the throat that is barely sore) will stop a cold developing.

Ferr. Phos.—for inflammation such as festering of a wounded finger—every half hour till it has subsided.

Kali. Phos.—one dose at bedtime, with another at hand 'in case' is almost unfailing in getting an over-excited or disturbed child (or myself) straight off to sleep.

Mag. Phos.—spasmodic pains, periods pains. Two or three half- or quarter-hourly doses sometimes in hot water very effective. (My teenage daughter finds no similar relief.)

Nat. Mur.—Two or three half-hourly doses will help depression and despondency.

Nat. Phos.—only two doses over half an hour will usually stop flatulence.

Silica—half-hourly doses have reduced the tight swollen symptoms of a stye on the eyelid and the condition has cleared up.'

Mrs D.T., Gloucester

'I have used your Combination J tablets for about two weeks. I had a very heavy cold, running nose and coughing. My condition has improved in that I feel better all round. I am still coughing a bit but I am not producing any phlegm (it was green). I have also found your C tablets most effective for dyspepsia.'

Mrs E.M., Londonderry

'I would just like to let you know of my recent experience with the above mentioned tissue salts (*Kali. Phos.*).

I have recently moved from Woking, Surrey to a tiny village in Rutland. Although I have been lucky in getting a job, the whole way of life and lack of close friends resulted in my becoming extremely anxious and apprehensive in everything. This is completely out of character and even though people have been very kind and helpful, things didn't improve. Eventually I began to lose concentration at work and had nothing but black gloomy thoughts. Rather than go to a GP and be told to 'buck up' or be given anti-depressants, I decided to try *Kali. Phos.* and took the required dose for 'chronic cases'.

Within a week I was back to my normal jolly self. Maybe this is psychological—even so, I shall keep some *Kali. Phos.* nearby just in case.'

Mrs P.B., Rutland

'I have been taking Combination E tablets regularly three times a day for just over two months and have found them helpful in relieving abdominal pain and discomfort due to diverticulitis, which I have had for about 2½ years.'

J.S.G., Somerset

'May I take this opportunity to thank you for your past prompt service and tell you what a help your remedies are for my husband and me for arthritis, rheumatism and the small daily ailments we have now we are 81 and 88 years old.'

Mrs N.H., Lancs.

'I feel I must write and tell you how much relief I have had since taking your combination tablets. I had been in considerable pain, with aching legs and couldn't sleep. Years ago, after having had an ulcer, I took a course of combination tablets and had relief so went back to them just a month ago. I am pleased to say I am able to get about and sleep normally now.'

Mrs D.H., Herts.

'I was recommended to your treatment some years ago by a friend who got them from London for me and, due to complicated circumstances, have not picked them up again for some time—having since moved, etc. However, my husband has recently had a recurrence of back pain and I gave him some of your Combination A for neuralgia/sciatica, etc., and he found quite a quick response—i.e. relief of pain and relaxation of pressure.

I have also had the rheumatism ones from time to time and found them very good.

However, I have now run out of both tablets and would like to have some 'by me'. Will you please advise where I can get them.'

Mrs P.W.M., Lincs.

INDEX

INDEX

For specific medical conditions readers are referred to pages 41–52.